PEGAN DIET:

Delicious, Quick & Easy to Make Recipes With 14-day Meal Plan for Healthy Lifestyle, Burn Fat & Lose Weight.

By

Talia Elliott

TABLE OF CONTENTS

Introduction 4

What is the pegan diet? 7

What does this tell you?..8

Responsible source of protein 9

Essentials of the Pegan diet....................... 10

Healthiest diet 10

Foods to eat while on the Pegan Diet 11

Pegan Diet, Food to Avoid....................................13

Are you confused about the pegan diet food selection?......15

DAY 1..17

Breakfast: PALEO STRAWBERRY COCONUT SMOOTHIE 17

Lunch: ROASTED RAINBOW VEGETABLE BOWL 18

Dinner: PAN-SEARED SALMON WITH KALE AND APPLE SALAD 22

DAY 2... 24

Breakfast: VEGETABLE VEGAN FRITTATA 24

Lunch: PALEO VEGGIE MUSHROOM BURGERS.................... 28

Dinner: 2 INGREDIENT CAULIFLOWER PALEO GNOCCHI.......31

DAY 3... 35

Breakfast: ONE-PAN EGGS WITH ASPARAGUS AND TOMATOES 35

Lunch: CASHEW CRUNCH SALAD WITH SESAME DRESSING 37

Dinner: INSTANT POT VEGAN PHO 39

DAY 4... 43

Breakfast: PALEO VEGAN PANCAKES 43

Lunch: Lemon Garlic Shrimp With Broccoli And Zucchini Noodles 45

Dinner: 3 INGREDIENT SWEET POTATO PIZZA CRUST.........48

DAY 5 .... **52**

Breakfast: RASPBERRY ALMOND OVERNIGHT OATS 52

LUNCH: MEAN GREEN DETOX SALAD 54

Dinner: THAI MANGO AVOCADO SALAD WITH GRILLED SWEET POTATOES 57

DAY 6 .... **60**

Breakfast: CREAMY GOLDEN MILK SMOOTHIE 60

Lunch: GARDEN EGG SALAD 63

Dinner: SURF AND TURF FOR TWO 65

DAY 7 .... **69**

Breakfast: EGGS BAKED IN TOMATOES 69

Lunch: CROWD-PLEASING VEGAN CAESAR SALAD 71

Dinner: JACKFRUIT BBQ PIZZA WITH A SWEET POTATO CRUST 75

DAY 8 .... **78**

Breakfast: SHEET PAN BREAKFAST FAJITAS........................ 78

Lunch: VEGAN LOADED SWEET POTATOES 80

Dinner: LENTIL SALAD WITH ROASTED VEGETABLES 83

DAY 9 .... **88**

Breakfast: SWEET POTATO HASH AND FRIED EGGS 88

Lunch: SHRIMP COBB SALAD WITH LEMON GARLIC VINAIGRETTE 92

Dinner: CHICKEN FAJITA STUFFED SPAGHETTI SQUASH 95

DAY 10 .... **99**

Breakfast: PUMPKIN COCONUT SMOOTHIE RECIPE 99

Lunch: CAULIFLOWER FRIED RICE 100

Dinner: SWEET AND SPICY STIR FRY WITH CHICKEN AND BROCCOLI 103

DAY 11 106

Breakfast: Aip Friendly Breakfast Porridge..................... 106

Lunch: PALEO BAKED ZUCCHINI FRITTERS 109

Dinner: VEGETABLE RATATOUILLE................................... 113

Day 12 117

Breakfast: MAPLE PECAN BANANA BREAKFAST BAKEt....... 117

Lunch: ROASTED BUTTERNUT SqUASH CAULIFLOWER SALAD 119

Dinner: MEDITERRANEAN CAULIFLOWER RICE 121

DAY 13 124

Breakfast: VEGAN SWEET POTATO BREAKFAST BOWL...... 124

Lunch: VEGAN ZUCCHINI PASTA ALFREDO........................ 125

Dinner: MEXICAN CORN QUINOA SALAD........................... 127

DAY 14 130

Breakfast: MANGO CHIA PUDDING 130

Lunch: CROCK POT PALEO HAMBURGER SOUP................. 131

Dinner: INSTANT POT SHORT RIBS.................................. 134

Conclusion 137

INTRODUCTION

The term Pegan Diet was postulated sometime in 2015 by one **Dr. Mark Hyman**; it's somewhat a new concept, though, so don't bother if you're hearing it for the first time. Like you have guessed, more people are beginning to learn about it recently based on the number of people searching for pegan related topics online.

At first, the idea alone may appear foolish to some, but as one expert in the pegan diet puts it, it's simply *"the meat-heavy Paleo diet combined with meat-shunning veganism."*

Indeed, many persons have expressed divergent views on what is allowed on the **Paleo diet,**whuch is based specifically on foods that predate agriculture.The same views have been expressed on the vegan diet that says no intake of living creatures' products.

And the pegan you now know is a combination of these two diet ideas. To be more specific, the pegan diet wants observers to maintain a healthy diet lifestyle that ensures the consumption of more than enough colorful vegetation. The diet includes organic, grass-fed, and sustainably produced poultry and eggs that Dr. Hyman describes as a portion quantity "condi-meats," referring to protein as a side dish rather than making it the major food.

Recall also that sustainably harvested seafood that is low in mercury, like salmon, oysters, or shrimps, and healthy fats available in nuts, avocados, etc., readily comes to mind.

Referring to the benefit of the Pegan Diet, **CookingLight** nutritionist **CarolynWilliams, Ph.D.RD** noted:

"What I think is positive about the Pegan diet is that it's another so-called 'clean eating' approach... There's an emphasis on whole foods, less processed foods, and real food, rather than foods with added sugars or added fat that may be less healthy. And I really like the emphasis on fruit and vegetable,... It's going to be lower in sodium than the typical American diet, and I like that it's a little more liberal than Paleo."

It is one of the trendiest eating plans right now, the pegan diet combines the paleo eating plan and vegan eating plan for a somewhat contradictory diet that boasts plenty of benefits. While the paleo diet has you eating like a cave(wo)man, the vegan diet has you eliminating all animal products.

Sound confusing? It kind of is, but it's working wonders for people. On the pegan diet, you can eat some meat, fish, and eggs, but it limits whole grains, dairy, and legumes.

WHAT IS THE PEGAN DIET?

The pegan diet is a dieting principle that adheres to the paleo and vegan diets, which is based on the idea that nutrient-dense, whole foods are capable of reducing inflammation, moderate blood sugar level, and as well provide optimal health.

Like many, you may have concluded that following the paleo and vegan, at the same time, will not be possible; this expert says it is quite understandable.

You may have read or heard certain persons talk about their personal experiences while on the Pegan Diet.How fascinating was it?Rather, did you find such stories a little odd?

I also have a contribution from back in the "good old days," as some use to say. I was purely on a vegan diet and later changed to a vegetarian diet.

But at some point again, I wanted something new, so I decided to switch to the Pegan Diet. I must confess, it indeed was confusing for me initially, owing to the fact that a low-carb and protein-rich diet was okay for me before then.

Yes, I actually started it out with a trial and error kind of method because I wasn't sure of the actual outcome, but I was hoping for something to come up. Did you hear me say I tried it for three weeks? Yes, I did, and then I saw the changes that I was looking for.

Pegan Diet is a special diet with a peculiar set of guidelines and is less restrictive than a paleo diet and the vegan diet.

It emphasizes more on eating vegetables and fruit and moderately consuming a certain amount of meat, fish, seeds, and nuts, with some legumes being inclusive.

Largely processed oils, sugars, and grains are not permitted, as a matter of principle, though an intake of a very small amount of this may not be an issue.

The pegan diet is not designed as a typical, short-term diet. Instead, it aims to be more sustainable so that you can follow it indefinitely.

What does this tell you?

The pegan diet, though standing on the paleo and vegan diets principles, still has its special rubric that is made in such a way as to encourage sustainability over a long period.

As a rule, those on pegan diets is hoping to consume fruits and vegetables up to 75%; and 25% of other foods primarily divided among eggs, meats; healthy fats, like nuts and seeds, including also certain legumes and gluten-free whole grains that you can take in limited quantities.

Responsible source of protein

While this diet principle encourages more plant-based foods, enough animal protein consumption is advised. Note also that as 75% of diets consist of vegetables and fruits, you're likely to have a reduced meat consumption compared to that of the average paleo diet, although more compared to any vegan diet.

This diet will not allow you to eat conventionally manufactured meats or eggs; rather, the emphasis is placed on grass-fed, pasture-raised foundations of beef, poultry, and pork; whole eggs too.

Low mercury content fish like wild salmon and sardines, in particular, is promoted as a better source of protein.

ESSENTIALS OF THE PEGAN DIET

Are you sure you're ready to start the pegan diet?Perhaps you have alerted your relatives (household members) about your newfound diet to prepare them for this carb-reduction diet? Let me not bother you with the headache, irritability, uncontrollable fatigue, and cravings often associated with removing carbs from one's diet. You could try creating a couple of days' worth of a meal plan, with a grocery inventory patterned to take care of the recipes you will need.

Healthiest diet

For those who want to know why the pegan diet is becoming popular in recent times, it will interest you to know that it's among the healthiest diets scientifically proven to be effective.

Just recently, a study came out suggesting the first five healthiest foods to include: the Low-carb, whole-food diet that is promoted mostly for people who want to lose weight and reduce the risk of disease infection for optimum health; the Mediterranean diet, the Paleo diet, the Vegan diet, and the Gluten-free diet.

Foods to eat while on the Pegan Diet

As you would soon find out, the pegan dietstrongly promotes those whole foods or those foods that do not undergo much or no processing at all before you eat them. As you have guessed already, that is why plants seem to have a bigger stake in the pegan diet.

As a matter of principle, you're advised to eat lots of plants as a primary food source: thus vegetables and fruits, amounting to 75% of your total food consumption within the period.

Low-glycemic **fruits and vegetables, like non-starchy vegetables**, berries, and the likes, are encouraged to reduce once blood sugar reaction.

A small quantity of starchy vegetables and sweet fruits is often permitted for people that have achieved a healthy blood sugar regulation before commencing the diet.

As stated earlier, the **healthy protein** source should be a major part of the remaining 25 % of your food consumption after removing 75% for fruits and vegetables.

Again, you're expected to maintain **minimally processed fats,**otherwise refers to as **healthy fats** from foods sources like:

The Nuts- excluding peanuts

The Seeds- excluding refined seed oils

The Avocados and the olives- including cold-pressed olive and avocado oils

The Coconut- unrefined coconut oil is also allowed

The Omega-3s- with emphasis on the low-mercury fish or algae

You may also consider pasture-raised meats and whole eggs for the fat content of your pegan diet.

You can take selected whole grains and legumes, especiallythe gluten-free whole grains and legumes but in a very small amount; the majority of this kind of food is prohibited because of their role in influencing blood sugar.

Grain intake is estimated not to exceed a 1/2 cup or 125 grams in every meal, just as legume is kept below 1 cup or 75 grams each meal, respectively.

Few grains and legumes that you may consider eating will include:

Black rice, millet, quinoa, teff, oats, and amaranth- for **grains**

Black beans, lentils, pinto beans, and chickpeas- for **legumes**

Diabetes patients or related medical condition patients that encourage poor blood sugar regulation should keep away from grains and legumes.

Bottom of Form

Pegan Diet, Food to Avoid

Those who want to go with the pegan diet should understand its principles and know those foods that are not allowed or at most are discouraged because of their nutritional content or relative response it evokes in the body.

Things like:

Sugar

Gluten

Dairy

Canola, soybean, corn oils, or grapeseed

Anything that has encountered certain chemical additives like pesticides, hormones, dyes, GMOs, artificial sweeteners, antibiotics, and preservatives, should not be consumed.

As a general Rule on this Diet, you're advised to at all times do the following:

Reduce starchy veggies in your meal, e.g., potatoes or the winter squash, to something less than ½ cup in a day while also consuming only the lower-sugar fruits like the berries and kiwi. If you must eat beans, it should be limited to something less than a cup daily.

Whole grains that do not have gluttons like teff, black rice, quinoa, and amaranth should also be eaten cautiously, with something less than ½ cup in each meal.

Once in a while, you may take honey or sugar in the form of maple syrup.

You may also eat once in a while grass-fed, organic dairy products like ghee or kefir. When there are no adverse result reports in terms of discomfort, milk product of sheep and goats may also be taken.

Every food taken should be modestly processed with a significant part of its natural content still intact.

Although pegan diet does not explicitly mention alcohol, the paleo diet forbids it.

Are you confused about the pegan diet food selection?

Well, a lot of persons on Pegan Diet say they'd literary have to check every label while shopping to effectively determine, for instance, the whole, organic or added-sugar-free items.

They're even more confused in ascertaining which among numerous choices are minimally processed foods; not to talk of knowing what the term addictive has to do with their choice, but then to answer these questions and many others Dr. Williams concludes by saying,

"There's no real definition of 'clean' and no real definition of 'processed,... Even if you buy cow's milk or raw chicken breasts, there's some sort of processing behind it. Even extra-virgin olive oil is technically processed. I try to steer people toward minimally processed, choosing foods as close to how they are in nature. When I look at the ingredients list, I think: If I were making this

at home, would it have these ingredients in it? I'm looking for chemicals or colorings or added sugars, more industrialized chemicals that aren't necessarily required for the food. They don't provide nutrients or play a key role in stabilizing the product."

You want to know what it tastes like? Why not try this 14days diet plans with full details!

DAY 1

Breakfast: PALEO STRAWBERRY COCONUT SMOOTHIE

This paleo strawberry coconut smoothie is sweet and creamy with no added sugar or dairy.

PREP TIME: 5 Minutes

TOTAL TIME: 5 Minutes

SERVINGS: 2 Servings

INGREDIENTS:

1 cup coconut milk
1 frozen banana sliced
2 cups frozen strawberries
1 teaspoon vanilla extract
1 scoop collagen peptides optional

INSTRUCTIONS:

Add all ingredients to high-speed blender and blend until smooth.

NOTES:

For vegan: omit protein powder or substitute with a vegan-friendly protein powder
For vegetarian: omit protein powder or substitute with a vegetarian protein powder

NUTRITION FACTS:

Calories: 346kcal | Carbohydrates: 27g | Protein: 8g | Fat: 24g | Saturated Fat: 21g | Sodium: 40mg | Potassium: 680mg | Fiber: 4g | Sugar: 14g | Vitamin A: 40IU | Vitamin C: 90.9mg | Calcium: 43mg | Iron: 4.5mg

Lunch: ROASTED RAINBOW VEGETABLE BOWL

Healthy, easy, and delicious roasted vegetable bowl with tahini dressing and hemp seeds! The perfect 30-minute plant-based meal for any time of the day!

PREP TIME: 5 Minutes

COOK TIME: 25 Minutes

TOTAL TIME   30 Minutes

SERVINGS: 2 Servings

INGREDIENTS:

Vegetables:

3-4 medium red or yellow baby potatoes (sliced into 1/4-inch rounds)
1/2 large sweet potato (skin on // sliced into 1/4-inch rounds)
2 large carrots (halved and thinly sliced)
1 medium beet (sliced into 1/8-inch rounds)
4 medium radishes (halved, or quartered if large)
2 Tbsp avocado or melted coconut oil (divided // if oil-free, sub water or vegetable broth)
1 tsp curry powder (divided)
1/2 tsp sea salt (divided)
1 cup cabbage (thinly sliced)
1 medium red pepper (thinly sliced)
1 cup broccolini (roughly chopped)
2 cups chopped collard greens or kale (organic when possible)

Toppings:

1 medium lemon (juiced // ~3 Tbsp or 45 ml as original recipe is written // divided)
2 Tbsp tahini (divided)
2 Tbsp hemp seeds (divided)
1/2 medium avocado (divided // optional)

INSTRUCTIONS:

Preheat oven to 400 degrees F (204 C) and line two baking sheets with parchment paper (or more baking sheets if increasing batch size).

To one baking sheet, add the potatoes, sweet potatoes, carrots, beets, and radishes and drizzle with half of the oil (or water), curry powder, and sea salt (as original recipe is written- 1 Tbsp (15 ml) oil (or water), 1/2 tsp curry powder, and 1/4 tsp sea salt). Toss to combine. Bake for a total of 20-25 minutes or until golden brown and tender.

To the second baking sheet, add the cabbage, bell pepper, and broccolini. Drizzle with with the remaining half of the oil (or water), curry powder, and sea salt (as original recipe is written- 1 Tbsp (15 ml) oil (or water), 1/2 tsp curry powder, and 1/4 tsp sea salt). Toss to combine.

When the potatoes/carrots hit the 10-minute mark, add the second pan to the oven and bake for a total of 15-20 minutes. In the last 5 minutes of baking, add the collard greens or kale to either pan and roast until tender and bright green.

To serve, divide vegetables between serving plates and garnish with avocado (optional) and season with lemon juice, tahini, hemp seeds, and another pinch of sea salt (optional). You could also garnish with any fresh herbs you have!

Best when fresh. Store leftovers covered in the refrigerator for 3-4 days. Reheat in a 350-degree F (176 C) oven or on the stovetop over medium heat until hot.

NOTES:

Nutrition information is a rough estimate without optional avocado.
For a salad version of this recipe, check out our 5-Minute Detox Salad!

Prep time does not indicate total hands-on prep time, but also includes prep completed while other items are cooking.

NUTRITIONFACTS:

Calories:	519
Carbohydrates:	59.2 g
Protein:	13.2 g
Fat:	28.4 g
Saturated Fat:	14.5 g
Trans Fat:	0 g

Cholesterol:	0 mg
Sodium:	518 mg
Fiber:	12.5 g
Sugar:	13.7 g

Dinner: PAN-SEARED SALMON WITH KALE AND APPLE SALAD

PREP TIME:	20 Minutes
TOTAL TIME:	30 Minutes
SERVINGS:	4 Servings

INGREDIENTS:

4 5-oz center-
cut salmon fillets (about 1" thick)
3 Tbsp fresh lemon juice
3 Tbsp olive oil
Kosher salt
1 bunch kale, ribs removed, leaves very thinly sliced (about 6 cups)
¼ cup dates
1 Honeycrisp apple
¼ cup finely grated pecorino
3 Tbsp toasted slivered almonds

Freshly ground black pepper
4 whole wheat dinner rolls

INSTRUCTIONS:

Bring the salmon to room temperature 10 minutes before cooking.

Meanwhile, whisk together the lemon juice, 2 tablespoons of the olive oil and 1/4 teaspoon salt in a large bowl. Add the kale, toss to coat and let stand 10 minutes.

While the kale stands, cut the dates into thin slivers and the apple into matchsticks. Add the dates, apples, cheese and almonds to the kale. Season with pepper, toss well and set aside.

Sprinkle the salmon all over with 1/2 teaspoon salt and some pepper. Heat the remaining 1 tablespoon oil in a large nonstick skillet over medium-low heat. Raise the heat to medium-high. Place the salmon, skin-side up in the pan. Cook until golden brown on one side, about 4 minutes. Turn the fish over with a spatula, and cook until it feels firm to the touch, about 3 minutes more.

Divide the salmon, salad and rolls evenly among four plates.

DAY 2

Breakfast: VEGETABLE VEGAN FRITTATA

This vegan vegetable frittata using a creamy tofu base is loaded with veggies. Perfect for a hearty breakfast/brunch and leftovers store well. Recipe adapted from PETA.

PREP TIME: 10 Minutes

COOK TIME: 50 Minutes

TOTAL TIME: 1 hour

SERVINGS: 6 Servings

INGREDIENTS:

1 tablespoon olive oil or ¼ cup water (for water saute)
2 medium potatoes, diced (with or without the skin)
1 small onion, diced
1 bell pepper, diced
1 zucchini, diced
2 cloves garlic, minced
handful grape tomatoes, halved or quartered
pinch of red pepper flakes, optional

mineral salt and pepper, to taste

for the blender/food processor:

1 package (16 oz) organic silken tofu (soft or firm), drained (no pressing needed)
¼ cup unsweetened non-dairy milk
2 heaping teaspoons cornstarch, arrowroot or tapioca flour
2 – 3 tablespoons nutritional yeast
1 teaspoon mustard (any kind) or ½ teaspoon mustard powder
1 ½ teaspoons dried tarragon, thyme or basil (or a combo)
½ teaspoon garlic powder
½ teaspoon salt
¼ teaspoon turmeric
⅛ teaspoon pepper (black or white)

INSTRUCTIONS

Preheat oven to 375 degrees F.
Saute: Heat oil in a pan over medium heat, saute potatoes for 5 minutes, add onion and cook an additional 5 minutes. Add bell pepper, zucchini and garlic, cook until softened. Add tomatoes and optional red pepper flakes, cook another minute or two. Season with salt and pepper to taste.

Tofu egg: In a food processor/blender, combine the remaining ingredients and process until smooth. Then taste for seasoning.

Assemble: Add the tofu mixture to the pan the vegetables cooked in and mix well. Spoon mixture into a lightly greased 9 inch round pie/quiche dish or springform pan. Level the top flat with the back of a spatula or spoon and make sure all edges are filled.

Bake: Place on the middle rack and bake for 35 – 45 minutes, frittata should be firm to the touch. If top starts to brown too much, cover with foil or small silpat. Remove and let cool for at least 10 minutes. If using a pie/quiche dish, loosen the edges of the frittata, place a plate over top and carefully flip so frittata falls onto the plate and serve (this step is optional).

This frittata is wonderful with sliced avocado and a little sriracha for heat.
Store: Leftovers can be stored in the refrigerator for 4 – 5 days. To keep longer, store in the freezer using freezer safe containers for up to 2 – 3 months.

NOTES:

I suggest using at least a 9-inch round dish or larger.

Nutritional information is calculated using water to saute, there is no oil accounted for.

Nutritional values are estimates only. See our full nutrition disclosure here.

NUTRITION FACTS:

Amount Per Serving

Calories 183

% Daily Value*

Total Fat 6.7g   9%

Saturated Fat 1g

Cholesterol 0mg   0%

Sodium 251.4mg   11%

Total Carbohydrate 18.1g   7%

Dietary Fiber 4.3g   15%

Sugars 2.6g

Protein 15.5g   31%

Lunch: PALEO VEGGIE MUSHROOM BURGERS

PREP TIME: 10 Minutes

COOK TIME: 40 Minutes

TOTAL TIME: 50 Minutes

INGREDIENTS:

1 teaspoon olive oil
16 ounces mushrooms, cut into 1/4 inch slices
1 red onion caramelized, cut into 1/4 inch slices
1 sweet potato, sliced thinly
1/4 cup walnuts, lightly toasted
1/4 teaspoon red pepper flakes
1/2 teaspoon Italian seasoning
1/4 teaspoon onion powder
1/4 teaspoon garlic powder
1/2 teaspoon ginger powder
3/4 cup almond flour
1 egg
1 teaspoon chia seeds
1/4 teaspoon sea salt, more to taste
1/4 teaspoon black pepper, more to taste

Toppings:

Tomato, sliced 1/4 inch thick
Red onion, sliced thinly
Pickles
Mustard
Ketchup

INSTRUCTIONS:

Pre-heat oven to 400 °F.
In a medium skillet over high heat, cook mushrooms and onions until caramelized. About 8-10 minutes.

Place sweet potato on a sheet-tray lined with parchment paper. Toss in a teaspoon of olive oil, one teaspoon sea salt, and one teaspoon pepper. Roast for 15-20 minutes, or until fork tender.

In a food processor add mushrooms, onions, 1 cup of the cooked sweet potato, walnuts, spices, almond flour, egg and chia seeds. Pulse a few times until just combined, make sure not to over process the mixture. There should be pea like sized bits of sweet potato.

Line a sheet tray with parchment paper and bring the oven temperature down to 350 °F.
Shape the sweet potato and mushroom mixture into 6 one-inch patties.

Bake for 30 minutes or until the patties are firm to touch. Let cool for 5 minutes and serve warm with toppings of choice!

RECIPENOTES

Use the extra sweet potato as a side-dish and serve them with this honey mustard sauce!

NUTRITIONFACTS:

Calories:	129
Sugar:	2.8g
Sodium:	102mg
Fat:	8.1g
Saturated Fat:	0.8g
Carbohydrates:	10g
Fiber:	3.8g
Protein:	6.5g
Cholesterol:	28mg

Dinner: 2 INGREDIENT CAULIFLOWER PALEO GNOCCHI

Homemade two ingredient cauliflower gnocchi. Easy, healthy, and delicious! An easy whole30 and paleo dinner that makes for easy meal prep.

COOK TIME: 40 Minutes

PREP TIME: 20 Minutes

SERVINGS: 4 Servings

INGREDIENTS:

Gnocchi
4 cups cauliflower minced
3/4 cup cassava flour
1/2 teaspoon sea salt optional

Sauce

1 can full fat canned coconut milk
4 cups spinach
2 large garlic cloves
2 tablespoons tapioca flour
salt and pepper to taste

INSTRUCTIONS

Heat oven to 425F.

Steam cauliflower for about five minutes until soft. Ring water out of cauliflower by putting it in a dish towel and squeezing the excess water out. The remaining cauliflower should measure out to about 1 1/2 cups.

In a food processor blend ingredients for gnocchi until smooth (you may have to add more or less cassava flour to get the dough to be kneadable). Separate dough into four equal parts and roll out into 3/4" diameter tubes on a surface dusted lightly with cassava flour. Cut the tubes of dough into 1" pieces.

Bring a large pot of water to a boil and drop gnocchi in. Once they have risen to the surface, remove, and drizzle lightly with olive oil.

Place gnocchi on a baking tray lined with parchment paper and lightly drizzled with olive oil. Bake on 425F for 20 minutes, then turn gnocchi over and bake for another 20 minutes until golden.

In a saucepan stir together ingredients for sauce (except spinach) and whisk continuously (or use a hand blender) until smooth and the sauce begins to thicken. If you overcook it, it will become too thick and gooey from the flour. Stir continuously to avoid clumping. Then remove from heat, add spinach, wilt it, then stir in gnocchi.

NUTRITIONFACTS:

Amount Per Serving

Calories 298   Calories from Fat 126

% DailyValue*

Total Fat 14g   22%

Saturated Fat 12g   60%

Polyunsaturated Fat 0.3g

Monounsaturated Fat 0.1g

Sodium 129mg   5%

Potassium 1062mg   30%

Total Carbohydrates 39g   13%

Dietary Fiber 8g   32%

Sugars 7g

Protein 7g   14%

Vitamin A	81%
Vitamin C2	17%
Calcium	10%
Iron	16%

DAY 3

Breakfast: ONE-PAN EGGS WITH ASPARAGUS AND TOMATOES

Raise your hand if you love eggs. Now raise the other if you hate cleaning up. Well, meet your new favorite recipe. This sheet-pan egg dish is basically the perfect meal, which you can serve for breakfast or dinner.

PREP TIME: 10 Minutes

COOK TIME: 20 Minutes

TOTAL TIME: 30 Minutes

SERVINGS: 4 Servings

INGREDIENTS:

2 pounds asparagus
1 pint cherry tomatoes
4 eggs
2 tablespoons olive oil
2 teaspoons chopped fresh thyme
Salt and pepper to taste

INSTRUCTIONS:

Preheat the oven to 400°F. Grease a baking sheet with non-stick cooking spray.
Arrange the asparagus and cherry tomatoes in an even layer on the baking sheet. Drizzle the olive oil over the vegetables; season with the thyme and salt and pepper to taste.

Roast in the oven until the asparagus is nearly tender and the tomatoes are wrinkled, 10 to 12 minutes.

Crack the eggs on top of the asparagus; season each with salt and pepper.

Return to the oven and bake until the egg whites are set, but the yolks are still jiggly, 7-8 minutes more.

To serve, divide the asparagus, tomatoes and eggs among four plates.

NUTRITION FACTS:

calories	158
fat	11g
carbs	13g

protein	11g
sugars	7g

Lunch: CASHEW CRUNCH SALAD WITH SESAME DRESSING

PREP TIME: 30 Minutes

TOTAL TIME: 30 Minutes

SERVINGS: 6–8 Servings

INGREDIENTS:

For the Salad:

1/2 head of green cabbage, finely shredded
1/2 head of purple cabbage, finely shredded
2 cups carrots, matchstick-cut or shredded
1 cup fresh cilantro, chopped
1/2 cup sliced green onion
2 cups cooked edamame (see notes)
1–2 cup roasted cashews (see notes)
2 cups crunchy chow mein noodles (optional)
chicken, shrimp, or any other protein you like

Dressing:

1/4 cup olive oil (you can use any other oil as well)
3 tablespoons white vinegar

2 tablespoons sesame oil – very important for flavor!
2 tablespoons sugar
1 teaspoon salt
a few shakes of garlic powder
optional: 1/4 cup Greek yogurt or mayo (more or less to taste)

INSTRUCTIONS:

Shake the dressing ingredients up in a jar until smooth. Add the Greek yogurt or mayo (optional just makes it more creamy) and shake again until smooth. YUM.

Toss all the salad ingredients together. Drizzle with dressing and serve!

NUTRITION FACTS:

Calories Per Serving: 337

% Daily Value

Total Fat 22.1g	28%
Cholesterol 0mg	0%
Sodium 606.9mg	26%
Total Carbohydrate 29.8g	11%

Dietary Fiber 5.3g	19%
Sugars 9.9g	
Protein 8.5g	17%
Vitamin A 292.4µg	32%
Vitamin C 42.3mg	47%

Dinner: INSTANT POT VEGAN PHO

This Vegan Pho soup recipe is a tasty combination of savory flavored broth along with traditional Vietnamese vegetables. Learn how to make vegan pho and season the broth with star anise, cloves and more.

PREP TIME:	10 Minutes
COOK TIME:	3 Minutes
ADDITIONAL TIME:	15 Minutes
TOTAL TIME:	28 Minutes
SERVINGS:	6 Servings

INGREDIENTS:

Fine mesh sieve

Pho bowls
Reusable chopsticks
Vietnamese Instant Pot cookbook
Vegan pho broth recipe
1 tablespoon olive oil
10 whole black peppercorns
3 whole star anise
1/2 teaspoon ground clove
1 tablespoon garlic
1 teaspoon ground ginger
1 cinnamon stick
1 white onion, quartered
2 (28-ounce) cans vegetable broth
1 1/2 cups shiitake mushrooms
1 baby bok choy
6 spring onions
1 teaspoon salt
8.8 ounce package thin rice noodles
Pho soup Toppings
Lime
Jalapeno
Spring onions/Chives
Cilantro

INSTRUCTIONS:

Place instant pot on sauté mode. Add in olive oil, black peppercorns, star anise, clove, garlic, ginger, and the cinnamon stick. Sauté about two minutes. Add in quartered onion and sauté another two minutes. Turn off sauté mode.

Pour in vegetable broth. Add in mushrooms. Add in spring onion bottoms reserving the chives for topping later. Pull the baby bok choy apart and wash. Add to pot. Add in salt and stir well.

Place lid onto the instant pot. Set valve to seal position. Press high pressure/pressure cook/manual button and set time to 1 minute. The broth will heat up as it comes to pressure.

Meanwhile, cook the rice noodles as direct on the stove. These have special instructions and shouldn't be made in the pot.

Once complete add the noodles to the pho. Serve with limes, jalapeno, cilantro, and any other toppings.

NUTRITIONFACTS:

Amount Per Serving

Calories	212
Total Fat	5g
Saturated Fat	1g
Trans Fat	0g

Unsaturated Fat	4g
Cholesterol	14mg
Sodium	1029mg
Carbohydrates	33g
Fiber	4g
Sugar	5g
Protein	11g

DAY 4

Breakfast: PALEO VEGAN PANCAKES

Paleo Vegan Pancakes are soft on the inside and slightly crispy on the outside. A scrumptious pancake that even those who follow an egg-free AND grain-free lifestyle can enjoy. Top with Roasted Strawberry Vanilla Bean Sauce for extra deliciousness.

PREP TIME: 15 Minutes

TOTAL TIME: 15 Minutes

SERVINGS: 4 Servings

INGREDIENTS:

1 cup almond flour
3/4 cup tapioca flour
1 Tbsp. baking powder
1/4 tsp. sea salt
2/3 cup unsweetened almond milk
2 tsp. apple cider vinegar
1 Tbsp. maple syrup
1 Tbsp. coconut oil, melted
1 tsp. pure vanilla extract

INSTRUCTIONS:

Combine all of the ingredients in a blender. Blend for a few seconds then stop blender and scrape sides and blend for a few seconds longer. You may also make the batter in a bowl however, blending does help to make these egg-free pancakes fluffier as stated above.

If needed, add additional liquid or flour in small increments (1/2 Tbsp. at a time) to achieve pancake batter consistency.

On medium/medium high heat pour batter on a greased skillet, about a scant 1/4 cup of batter per pancake.

Flip when pancakes begin to bubble or spatula easily slips under pancake. Continue to cook until golden brown on both sides.

Allow pancakes to cool slightly before enjoying. Top the desired toppings such as Roasted Strawberry Vanilla Bean Sauce and nut butter.

NOTES

recipe, please rewrite the recipe in your unique words and link back to the source recipe here on The Real Food Dietitians. Thank you!

NUTRITION FACTS:

Serving Size: 1/4 calories: 283 sugar: 4g Sodium: 200mg fat: 18g carbohydrates: 29g fiber: 3g Protein: 6g

Lunch: Lemon Garlic Shrimp With Broccoli And Zucchini Noodles

PREP TIME:	10 Minutes
COOK TIME:	5 Minutes
TOTAL TIME:	15 Minutes
SERVINGS:	2 Servings

INGREDIENTS:

1 tablespoon ghee or grass fed unsalted butter
1 tablespoon extra-virgin olive oil
4 garlic cloves, minced
½ cup chicken or vegetable broth or white wine
1/2 teaspoon Celtic sea salt, or to taste
⅛ teaspoon crushed red pepper flakes, or to taste
Freshly ground black pepper

6–8 ounces wild large or extra-large shrimp, peeled and deveined with tails on (fresh or frozen and thawed), I used 9 shrimp.
2 cups broccoli florets (size the broccoli so it will cook in the same amount of time as shrimp)*
4 cups spiralized zucchini noodles (optional "sweat" with 1/2 teaspoon Celtic sea salt)*
2 tablespoons lemon juice
1/4 cup chopped parsley
Vegan parmesan or parmesan cheese (optional)

INSTRUCTIONS:

In a large skillet, melt ghee or butter with olive oil. Add garlic and sauté on medium low until fragrant, about 1 minute.

Add broth, salt, red pepper flakes and a large pinch of black pepper and bring to a simmer.
Simmer the stock for about one minute to develop flavors.

Add shrimp and broccoli. Sauté on medium turning the shrimp once, until they just turn pink and the broccoli is bright green, 2 to 4 minutes depending upon their size.

Add the zucchini noodles, parsley and lemon.
Toss the noodles with the shrimp so they are coated with the garlic-lemon sauce. Heat just

until warmed through, 1 minute. (Do not overcook or the zucchini noodles will become mushy.)

Sprinkle with parsley and vegan or regular parmesan.

NOTES:

Recipe can be made without broccoli, just the shrimp and zucchini noodles.

If your zucchini are medium to large I recommend "sweating" the spiralized zucchini before adding them to the pan. To "sweat" the zucchini noodles, place them in a colander, then place the colander in the sink or over a bowl. Sprinkle with 1/2 teaspoon salt and toss. Allow them to sit for about 20 minutes – the longer it sits, the more water is drawn out. After the 20 minutes or longer, squeeze all the water out with a kitchen towel.

NUTRITIONFACTS:

Calories Per Serving: 284

% DailyValue

Total Fat 14.7g   19%

Cholesterol 154.6mg	52%
Sodium 798.5mg	35%
Total Carbohydrate 17.3g	6%
Dietary Fiber 5.3g	19%
Sugars 8.3g	
Protein 25.9g	52%
Vitamin A 133.1µg	15%
Vitamin C 143.3mg	59%

Dinner: 3 INGREDIENT SWEET POTATO PIZZA CRUST

PREP TIME: 20 Minutes

COOK TIME: 40 Minutes

TOTAL TIME: 1 hour

SERVINGS: 2 Servings(2 individual pan pizzas or 1 crust that can be divided

INGREDIENTS:

One medium sweet potato, peeled
2/3 cup rolled oats

One egg
1/2 teaspoon salt
a pinch of garlic powder
One tablespoon olive oil

INSTRUCTIONS:

Preheat oven to 400 degrees. Pulse the sweet potato and oats through the food processor until very fine. Add the egg and garlic powder and salt; pulse again to mix. The mixture should resemble a loose dough or thick batter.

Transfer to a parchment lined baking sheet or round pizza pan. Press into crusts and shape with your hands – you can either make two smaller crusts (you'll get more crispy edge surface area) or one larger crust. Crusts should be about 1/4 to 1/2 inch thick.

Bake for 25-30 minutes, until the top is dry to the touch. Remove from oven, let cool, and invert back onto the pan with the dry side facing down. Peel the parchment very gently off the top layer and brush with olive oil. Bake for another 5-10 minutes to get a nice crispy top.

Top with your favorite pizza toppings and pop back into the oven to melt the cheese! Voila.

NOTES:

When you peel the parchment paper off, the crust will want to stick to the parchment paper. Just do this slowly and carefully – it should work fine, and even if a few little tiny bits of crust come off with the parchment, your crust will still hold together.

If it's really an issue, stick it back in the oven for a few minutes with the parchment paper ON TOP to dry it out. This will make it easier to pull off. If the hand-holdable factor is of importance to you, I would let the crust cool and dry out a little bit before baking.

High-moisture toppings such as tomato sauce and mozzarella cheese can really do a number on the hand-holdability of this crust and might require some fork action. We found the BBQ Chicken pizza toppings (BBQ sauce, chicken, cheese, red onion, cilantro) were the most likely to give us a crust that was still hand-holdable even after baking.

NUTRITIONFACTS:

Serving Size: Half Pizza

Calories Per Serving: 258

% Daily Value

Total Fat 9.4g   12%

Cholesterol 93mg   31%

Sodium 654.4mg   28%

Total Carbohydrate 32.7g   12%

Dietary Fiber 4.8g   17%

Sugars 2.9g

Protein 7.8g   16%

Vitamin A 511.5µg   57%

DAY 5

Breakfast: RASPBERRY ALMOND OVERNIGHT OATS

PREP TIME:	5 Minutes
TOTAL TIME:	5 Minutes
SERVINGS:	1 Servings

INGREDIENTS:

½ cup old-fashioned oats
1 cup almond milk
¼ cup almond yogurt
2 tablespoons chia seeds
1 tablespoon maple syrup
½ cup raspberries
2 tablespoons almond butter
2 tablespoons sliced almonds

INSTRUCTIONS:

In a pint-sized mason jar or medium sized bowl, add the rolled oats, almond yogurt, almond milk, chia seeds and maple syrup. Stir well so that the oats are coated with the mixture and the chia seeds don't clump up together.

Cover the container and place in the fridge overnight for at least 12 hours.
The next day, give the oats a quick stir and add a splash of almond milk to thin the mixture if needed.

Then top with a scoop of almond butter, raspberries, sliced almonds and whatever additional oatmeal toppings you enjoy most.

NOTES:

This recipe is vegan, gluten free and dairy free!
Try stirring the almond butter into the no cook oatmeal when preparing for a rich and satisfying taste.

Enjoy within 5 days of preparation to ensure the ingredients do not spoil.

NUTRITIONFACTS:

Amount Per Serving: Calories: 539 Total Fat: 22g saturated Fat: 2g Trans Fat: 0g unsaturated Fat: 18g Cholesterol: 0mg Sodium: 30mg Carbohydrates: 76g Fiber: 16g Sugar: 28g Protein: 14g

LUNCH: MEAN GREEN DETOX SALAD

PREP TIME:	30 Minutes
COOK TIME:	30 minutes
Total Time:	1 hour
SERVINGS:	4 servings

INGREDIENTS:

Lemon Tahini Dressing:

2 tablespoons tahini sesame seed paste
2 tablespoons olive oil
1 teaspoon low sodium soy sauce or tamari
juice + zest from 1 lemon use only half of the zest
2 cloves garlic grated
2 teaspoons fresh ginger grated
salt + pepper to taste

Salad:

2 cups cooked chickpeas
1 cup unsweetened flaked coconut
2 tablespoon low sodium soy sauce or tamari
2 tablespoons sesame oil
1/4 teaspoon cayenne pepper

4 cups Tuscan kale roughly torn
2 cups fresh broccoli florets
1/4 head purple cabbage shredded
1/2 cup fresh parsley + cilantro roughly chopped
hemp seeds + chia seeds for topping
2 red grapefruits segmented
2 ripe but firm avocados sliced or chopped

VeganParmesan:

1/2 cup raw pine nuts
2 teaspoons raw sesame seeds
1 tablespoon nutritional yeast
salt to taste

INSTRUCTIONS

Lemon Tahini Dressing:

Add all the ingredients to a bowl and whisk until combined. Taste and adjust salt + pepper to your liking. Alternately you can add the ingredients to a blender or food processor and blend until smooth. The dressing can be made a week in advance and stored in the fridge until ready to use.

Salad:

Preheat the oven to 425 degrees F.

Spread the chickpeas out on a towel and dry them completely. Add the chickpeas and coconut to a baking sheet and toss with the soy sauce, sesame oil and cayenne pepper.

Toss well to evenly coat. Roast for 20 minutes and then stir the chickpeas around and roast another 10 minutes or until the chickpeas are browned and the coconut is dark brown. Remove from the oven. Save any leftovers for snacking on later!

Add the kale to a large bowl and drizzle with 1 teaspoon olive oil and a big pinch of salt. Using your hands, massage the kale for 2-3 minutes until the kale is well coated and has slightly softened.

To the bowl add the broccoli, cabbage, parsley, and cilantro. Toss well. Add the dressing and continue to toss until all the veggies are coated. Add the grapefruit segments and avocado. Gently toss to combine. At this point, you can cover and store the salad in the fridge for up to 24 hours or continue on with the recipe.

Divide the salad into bowls. Top with the crunchy coconut chickpeas and the vegan parmesan cheese (recipe below) and a sprinkle of chia + hemp seeds. EAT!!

VeganParmesan:

In a food processor or blender, combine the pine nuts, sesame seeds, nutritional yeast and a pinch of salt. Processor until you have fine crumbs that resemble parmesan cheese. Taste and season with more salt if desired. The vegan parmesan can be made a week in advance and stored in the fridge until ready to use.

Dinner: THAI MANGO AVOCADO SALAD WITH GRILLED SWEET POTATOES

PREP TIME: 10 Minutes

COOK TIME: 10 Minutes

SERVINGS: 4 Servings

INGREDIENTS:

1 medium Sweet Potato, peeled and sliced 1/4 inch thick, 250g

1 tablespoon Coconut Oil, melted

1 cup Mango, about 1 mango or 180g

1 large Avocado, cubed, 120g

2/3 cup Cucumber, diced

1/4 cup Fresh Mint, thinly sliced and lightly packed

1/4 cup Fresh Cilantro, diced and packed

Sea Salt
For the Sauce:
4 teaspoons Fresh Lime Juice
2 teaspoons Fish Sauce, Paleo-friendly

INSTRUCTIONS:

Preheat your grill to high heat. Toss the sweet potato slices in the coconut oil and grill for 3-4 minutes per side, or until nice grill marks form. Once cool enough to handle, slice them into small cubes and add them into a large bowl.

Add in the mango, avocado, cucumber, mint and cilantro and stir until combined.

Mix the lime juice and fish sauce in a small bowl and pour over the salad. Toss to combine, and season to taste with salt.
DEVOUR!

NUTRITIONFACTS:

Amount Per Serving

Calories from Fat 76   Calories 156

% DailyValue*

Total Fat 10g   15%

Saturated Fat 4g   18%

Sodium 246mg   10%

Total Carbohydrate 17g   6%

Dietary Fiber 5g   6%

Sugars 6g   3%

DAY 6

Breakfast: CREAMY GOLDEN MILK SMOOTHIE

All of the delicious taste and health perks of golden milk in smoothie form! Just 7 ingredients, 1 blender, and 5 minutes required. Creamy, naturally sweet, subtly spiced, and packed with turmeric!

PREP TIME: 5 Minutes

TOTAL TIME: 5 Minutes

SERVINGS: 1 Serving

INGREDIENTS:

SMOOTHIE

1 cup banana* (ripe, sliced, and frozen)
1 cup light coconut milk or almond milk (or store-bought // use full-fat coconut for creamier smoothie)
1/2 tsp ground turmeric (preferred flavor over fresh)
1 Tbsp fresh ginger (plus more to taste)
1 Dash ground cinnamon
1 Dash black pepper

1 Dash ground nutmeg
1 Dash ground clove and cardamom (optional // for more warmth + spice)
1/4 cup fresh carrot juice* (optional // for color, added sweetness + balances banana flavor // or sub 1 small carrot!)

For Serving Optional

1 Tbsp Hemp seeds

INSTRUCTIONS:

Add banana, coconut milk, turmeric, ginger, cinnamon, black pepper, and nutmeg to a high-speed blender and blend on high until creamy and smooth. If including, add cardamom, clove, and fresh carrot juice at this time (optional).

If too thick, thin with more coconut milk or water. If too thin, thicken with ice (or more frozen banana, though it will add more sweetness).

Taste and adjust flavor as needed, adding more cinnamon for warmth, black pepper for spice, ginger for "zing," turmeric for earthiness / more intense color, or banana for sweetness. Adding carrot juice will also add sweetness and more intense orange/yellow hue.

Divide between serving glasses (ours are from West Elm) and enjoy immediately. Keep leftovers in the refrigerator for 24 hours. Freeze leftovers by pouring into an ice cube tray and use for future smoothies (either this smoothie or others you'd like to infuse with a golden milk flavor).

NOTES:

If you're trying to avoid/sub banana, we'd recommend using the recommended amount of carrot juice, swap the banana for the same amount of cauliflower, and add some vanilla protein powder for sweetness.

Make carrot juice in a juicer, buy at the store, or add 1 raw or cooked carrot to the smoothie to a similar effect.

Nutrition information is a rough estimate based on full recipe calculated with light (canned) coconut milk and without optional ingredients.

NUTRITIONFACTS:

Calories:	295
Carbohydrates:	43.7 g
Protein:	3.5 g

Fat:	13.9 g
Saturated Fat:	11.6 g
Polyunsaturated Fat:	0.67 g
Monounsaturated Fat:	0.54 g
Trans Fat:	0 g
Cholesterol:	0 mg
Sodium:	23.3 mg
Potassium:	1104 mg
Fiber:	4.6 g
Sugar:	17 g
Vitamin A:	88.84 IU
Vitamin C:	15.14 mg
Calcium:	57.59 mg
Iron:	8.84 mg

Lunch: GARDEN EGG SALAD

TOTAL TIME:	25 Minutes
ACTIVE TIME:	10 Minutes

SERVINGS: 4 Servings

INGREDIENTS:

6 large eggs
1/2 cup low-fat mayonnaise
2 tablespoons whole-grain mustard
Kosher salt and freshly ground black pepper
2 scallions (white and green), thinly sliced,
1 rib celery, minced, scant 1/2 cup
2 radishes, grated on the large holes of a box grater
8 romaine lettuce leaves
1 cup pea or other sprouts

INSTRUCTIONS:

Put the eggs in a saucepan with enough cold water to cover. Bring to a boil, cover, and remove from the heat. Set aside for 12 minutes. Drain the eggs and roll them between your palm and the counter to crack the shell, then peel under cool running water.

Dice the eggs. Combine the eggs with mayonnaise, mustard and season with the salt and pepper. Stir in the scallions, celery, and radish.

Divide the egg salad among the lettuce leaves, top with the sprouts and roll up. Serve 2 rolls per serving.

NUTRITIONFACTS:

Per Serving

Calories	266
Total Fat	17 grams
Saturated Fat	4 grams
Cholesterol	290 milligrams
Sodium	561 milligrams
Carbohydrates	14 grams
Dietary Fiber	3 grams
Protein	13 grams
Sugar	3 grams

Dinner: SURF AND TURF FOR TWO

This is a simple way to make a special dinner any night of the week. You probably have most of the ingredients in your pantry already. Serve shrimp alongside steaks with your favorite sides.

PREP TIME: 15 Minutes

COOK TIME: 15 Minutes

ADDITIONAL: 15 Minutes

TOTAL: 45 mins

SERVINGS: 2 Servings

INGREDIENTS:

1 tablespoon olive oil
1 tablespoon butter, melted
1 tablespoon finely minced onion
1 tablespoon white wine
1 teaspoon Worcestershire sauce
1 teaspoon lemon juice
1 teaspoon dried parsley
1 teaspoon seafood seasoning (such as Old Bay®)
1 clove garlic, minced
⅛ teaspoon freshly ground black pepper
12 medium shrimp, peeled and deveined
2 (4 ounce) filet mignon steaks
2 teaspoons olive oil
1 teaspoon steak seasoning

INSTRUCTIONS:

Whisk 1 tablespoon olive oil, butter, onion, wine, Worcestershire sauce, lemon juice, parsley, seafood seasoning, garlic, and black pepper together in a bowl; add shrimp. Toss to coat evenly. Cover bowl with plastic wrap and refrigerate for flavors to blend, at least 15 minutes.

Preheat an outdoor grill for medium-high heat and lightly oil the grate. Coat steaks with 2 teaspoons olive oil; sprinkle with steak seasoning.

Cook steaks until they are beginning to firm and have reached your desired doneness, 5 to 7 minutes per side. An instant-read thermometer inserted into the center should read 140 degrees F (60 degrees C). Transfer steaks to a platter and loosely tent with a piece of aluminum foil.

Remove shrimp from marinade and grill until they are bright pink on the outside and the meat is no longer transparent in the center, 2 to 3 minutes per side.

NOTES:

For thick steaks and medium doneness, grill over high heat 6 minutes on first side, 4 minutes on second side, or broil 3 inches from heat source, 8 minutes first side and 6 minutes on second. Steaks and shrimp can also be cooked stove-top in a heavy skillet with a coating of olive oil.

NUTRITIONFACTS:

Per Serving: 444 calories; protein 26.9g; carbohydrates 2.7g; fat 35.2g; cholesterol 165.9mg; sodium 925.6mg.

DAY 7

Breakfast: EGGS BAKED IN TOMATOES

PREP TIME:	25 Minutes
COOK TIME:	20 Minutes
TOTAL TIME:	45 Minutes
SERVINGS:	4 Servings

INGREDIENT:

2 tablespoons olive oil

8 medium tomatoes

8 large eggs

¼ cup milk

¼ cup grated Parmesan cheese

Salt and freshly ground black pepper

4 tablespoons chopped fresh herbs (like parsley, thyme, rosemary or a mixture)

INSTRUCTIONS:

Preheat the oven to 375°F. Grease a large, oven-safe skillet with the olive oil.

Using a small paring knife, cut around the stems of the tomatoes and remove them. Use a spoon to scoop out all the insides of the tomatoes. (Reserve the insides and use them to make tomato sauce or salsa.)

Arrange the tomato shells snugly in the prepared skillet. Crack an egg into each tomato. Top each egg with 1 tablespoon milk and 1 tablespoon Parmesan. Season each egg with salt and pepper. Bake until the tomatoes are tender, the egg whites are set and the yolks are still a little jiggly, 15 to 17 minutes. Let cool 5 minutes and then garnish with the fresh herbs. Serve immediately

NUTRITIONFACTS:

calories	288
fat	19g
carbs	12g
protein	18g
sugars	8g

Lunch: CROWD-PLEASING VEGAN CAESAR SALAD

PREP TIME:	45 Minutes
COOK TIME:	35 Minutes
SERVINGS:	6 Servings

INGREDIENTS:

For the Roasted Chickpea Croutons:

1 (14-ounce/398 mL) can chickpeas (or 1 1/2 cups cooked), drained and rinsed
1 teaspoon (5 mL) extra-virgin olive oil
1/2 teaspoon fine grain sea salt
1/2 teaspoon garlic powder
1/8 to 1/4 teaspoon cayenne pepper (optional)

For the Caesar Dressing (makes 3/4-1 cup):

1/2 cup raw cashews, soaked overnight
1/4 cup (60 mL) water
2 tablespoons (30 mL) extra-virgin olive oil
1 tablespoon (15 mL) lemon juice
1/2 tablespoon (7.5 mL) Dijon mustard
1/2 teaspoon garlic powder
1 small garlic clove (you can add another if you like it super potent)

1/2 tablespoon (7.5 mL) vegan Worcestershire sauce (I use Wizard's gluten-free brand)

2 teaspoons capers

1/2 teaspoon fine grain sea salt and pepper, or to taste

For the Nut and Seed Parmesan Cheese:

1/3 cup raw cashews

2 tablespoons hulled hemp seeds

1 small garlic clove

1 tablespoon nutritional yeast

1 tablespoon (15 mL) extra-virgin olive oil

1/2 teaspoon garlic powder

fine grain sea salt, to taste

For the lettuce:

1 small/medium bunch lacinato kale, destemmed (5 cups chopped)

2 small heads romaine lettuce (10 cups chopped)

INSTRUCTIONS:

Soak cashews in a bowl of water overnight, or for at least a few hours. Drain and rinse.

Roast chickpea croutons: Preheat oven to 400°F (200°C). Drain and rinse chickpeas. Place chickpeas in a tea towel and rub dry (it's okay if some skins fall off). Place onto large rimmed baking sheet. Drizzle on oil and roll around to coat. Sprinkle on the garlic powder, salt, and optional cayenne.

Toss to coat. Roast for 20 minutes at 400°F (200°C), then gently roll the chickpeas around in the baking sheet. Roast for another 10 to 20 minutes, until lightly golden. They will firm up as they cool.

Prepare the dressing: Add the cashews and all other dressing ingredients (except salt) into a high-speed blender, and blend on high until the dressing is super smooth. You can add a splash of water if necessary to get it blending. Add salt to taste and adjust other seasonings, if desired. Set aside.

Prepare the Parmesan cheese: Add cashews and garlic into a mini food processor and process until finely chopped. Now add in the rest of the ingredients and pulse until the mixture is combined. Salt to taste.

Prepare the lettuce: Destem the kale and then finely chop the leaves. Wash and dry in a salad spinner. Place into extra large bowl. Chop up the romaine into bite-sized pieces. Rinse and then spin dry. Place into bowl along with kale. You should have roughly 5 cups chopped kale and 10 cups chopped romaine.

Assemble: Add dressing onto lettuce and toss until fully coated. Season with a pinch of salt and mix again. Now sprinkle on the roasted chickpeas and the Parmesan cheese. Serve immediately.

TIPS:

Be sure to check the label to ensure your Worcestershire Sauce is gluten-free (if necessary) as not many are. I use Wizard`s Gluten-Free Organic Worcestershire Sauce.

The dressing thickens when chilled, so be sure to leave it at room temperature to soften before use.

NUTRITIONFACTS:

Calories 310 calories | Total Fat 17 grams

Saturated Fat 2.5 grams | Sodium 460 milligrams | Total Carbohydrates 29 grams

Fiber 9 grams | Sugar 4 grams | Protein 12 grams

Dinner: JACKFRUIT BBQ PIZZA WITH A SWEET POTATO CRUST

Jackfruit BBQ Pizza with a Sweet Potato Crust - Shredded jackfruit mixed in a homemade BBQ sauce along with sliced red onions and cilantro | Paleo + Vegan + Nut Free

PREP TIME: 15 minutes

COOK TIME: 15 minutes

TOTAL TIME   30 minutes

SERVINGS: 8 Slice

INGREDIENTS:

Pizza Crust:

1 sweet potato pizza crust

Bbq Sauce:

1/2 cup tomato sauce/passata, *see notes
1 tablespoon tomato paste
2 tablespoons coconut sugar
1 tablespoon molasses
1 tablespoon apple cider vinegar
1 tablespoon chili powder
1 teaspoon onion powder

1 teaspoon salt
1 teaspoon garlic powder
3/4 teaspoon paprika
1/2 teaspoon mustard powder
1 tablespoon chipotle paste, optional

Toppings:

1 cup jackfruit from a can in water
1/4 cup red onion, sliced
fresh cilantro, for topping

INSTRUCTIONS

Prep the sweet potato crust.

Bbq sauce & jackfruit:

Add everything to a small or medium sauce pot and whisk together over a medium low heat. Let simmer for 5 minutes. Measure

Drain and rinse jackfruit and then start breaking up the chunks into small pieces. You can use a fork or potato masher here to mash it all up but I find it easier to pull apart larger chunks with my fingers.

Stir in the broken up jackfruit into the remaining BBQ sauce and cook on a low heat for a few minutes.

Top pizza with jackfruit in BBQ sauce and sliced red onions. Bake at 400°F/205°C for 10 minutes.

Top with fresh cilantro and serve!

NUTRITIONFACTS:

Amount Per Serving: CALORIES: 146SATURATED FAT: 1gSODIUM: 589mgCARBOHYDRATES: 25gFIBER: 3gSUGAR: 5gPROTEIN: 2g

DAY 8

Breakfast: SHEET PAN BREAKFAST FAJITAS

PREP TIME:	15 Minutes
COOK TIME:	25 Minutes
TOTAL TIME:	40 Minutes
SERVINGS:	4 Servings

INGREDIENTS:

1 red bell pepper, thinly sliced
1 orange bell pepper, thinly sliced
1 green bell pepper, thinly sliced
2 tablespoons olive oil
1 tablespoon chili powder
1 tablespoon freshly squeezed lime juice
3 cloves garlic, minced
1 1/2 teaspoons ground cumin
1 teaspoon ground paprika
1/4 teaspoon onion powder
Kosher salt and freshly ground black pepper, to taste
6 large eggs
1 avocado, halved, peeled, seeded and sliced

1/4 cup chopped fresh cilantro leaves

INSTRUCTIONS:

Preheat oven to 400 degrees F. Lightly oil a baking sheet or coat with nonstick spray.

Place bell peppers in a single layer onto the prepared baking sheet. Stir in olive oil, chili powder, lime juice, garlic, cumin, paprika and onion powder, and gently toss to combine; season with salt and pepper, to taste.

Place into oven and bake until tender, about 12-15 minutes.

Remove from oven and create 6 wells. Add eggs, gently cracking the eggs throughout and keeping the yolk intact; season with salt and pepper, to taste.

Place into oven and bake until the egg whites have et, an additional 8-12 minutes.

Serve immediately, garnished with avocado and cilantro, if desired.

Lunch: VEGAN LOADED SWEET POTATOES

These vegan loaded sweet potatoes are sure to become a weeknight favorite. It's super simple to whip up and makes for filling plant-based dinner with black beans, corn, and avocado-lime topping.

PREP TIME: 10 Minutes

COOK TIME: 45 Minutes

TOTAL TIME: 55 Minutes

SERVINGS: 4 Servings

INGREDIENTS:

4 sweet potatoes
1/2 tablespoon olive oil
For the Filling:
1 tablespoon olive oil
1/2 cup chopped red onion (~1/2 small red onion)
1/2 bell pepper, chopped
1 tablespoon taco seasoning
2 cloves garlic, minced
1 (15 oz) can black beans, drained and rinsed
1/3 cup salsa
3/4 cup frozen (or fresh) corn

For the Avocado Topping:

1 avocado
1 jalapeno, seeds and stems removed (use 1/2 to make it less spicy)
1 clove garlic
1 green onion
2 tablespoons water (More to thin if desired)
Juice from 1 lime
Sea salt, to taste

INSTRUCTIONS:

Preheat the oven to 400 degrees Fahrenheit.

Wash sweet potatoes and poke a few times with a fork. Place on a baking sheet. Drizzle with oil and use your hands to make sure each potato is evenly coated in oil. Bake for 45-55 minutes or until potatoes are easily pierced with a fork. Set aside.

While the potatoes bake, add the olive oil and onions and pepper to a non-stick skillet over medium-high heat. Sautés until onions are translucent. Stir in the taco seasoning and garlic and sauté for 1 minute.

Stir in the black beans, salsa, corn, and ~1/4 teaspoon sea salt. Cook for 2-3 minutes. Taste and add more salt if needed. Set aside.

Add all of the avocado topping ingredients to a food processor and blend until smooth. I prefer a thick sauce that I can dollop on the potatoes, but you can add more water (1 tablespoon at a time) to make it thinner if you prefer.

To assemble, cut potatoes in half lengthwise and use fork to fluff insides. Top with 1/4 black bean filling and add a dollop of avocado topping. Garnish with sliced jalapeños, chopped red onion, and cilantro if desired.

NUTRITION FACTS:

Calories:	325 kcal
Sugar:	4 g
Sodium:	355 mg
Fat:	13 g
Saturated Fat:	2 g
Unsaturated Fat:	11 g
Trans Fat:	0 g
Carbohydrates:	43.5 g
Fiber:	14 g

Protein: 11.5 g

Cholesterol: 0 mg

Dinner: LENTIL SALAD WITH ROASTED VEGETABLES

PREP TIME: 10 Minutes

COOK TIME: 35 Minutes

TOTAL TIME: 45 Minutes

SERVINGS: 6 SERVINGS

INGREDIENTS:

3/4 cup french green or black beluga lentils
1 head cauliflower
1 lb. carrots*
2 red onions
2 small fennel bulbs or 1 large
1/2 cup pistachios*

Marinade/Dressing

1/3 cup olive oil
1/4 cup apple cider vinegar
1 Tablespoon pure maple syrup
2 teaspoons cinnamon
1 teaspoon cumin

1/2 teaspoon allspice
1/2 teaspoon turmeric
1/2 teaspoon ground ginger
1/2 teaspoon coarse sea salt
1/8 teaspoon cayenne
Garnish
1/3 cup golden raisins*
Fronds from the fennel
Something green: either chopped fresh parsley or stacked and julienned collard greens or lacinato kale.

INSTRUCTIONS:

Preheat oven to 400

PREPARE VEGGIES: Cut cauliflower into florets. Peel carrots and cut into thick circles. Cut onion through the root end and then into wedges or thin slices or a combo. Trim fennel fronds and save for garnish; cut through the center and then into 1/2" wedges. Place all in large bowl.

MAKE MARINADE: whisk together olive oil, vinegar and maple syrup until emulsified. Sprinkle in spices and mix again.

Pour 3/4 marinade over veggies and toss until evenly coated. Arrange in single layer on rimmed baking tray. You may need two trays to give them enough room to nicely brown. Roast for 35 minutes, until golden brown and tender.

Meanwhile, prepare lentils*. Rinse well and then place in a small saucepan with 3 cups water. Bring to boil and then turn down to simmer and cook for 16 minutes. You want tender, not mushy lentils. Drain and place in bowl that veggies were mixed in.

Pour remaining dressing/marinade over lentils and mix well. When veggies are done, add to bowl along with raisins and mix.

Arrange on platter: OPTIONAL: place thinly sliced greens (lacinato kale or collard greens) on bottom of platter and then veggie mix. Top with fennel fronds, a sprinkle of salt + pepper and more nuts or raisins as desired.

Roasted Veggies and lentils will stay good in the fridge for up to a week.

NOTES:

CARROTS: 1 lb. carrot is approximately five large carrots, or eight smaller carrots.
PISTACHIOS: For nut allergies, substitute with sunflower or pumpkin seeds.

RAISINS: Substitute any unsulfered and unsweetened dried fruit like cranberries or apricots for the chewy texture.

LENTILS: Directions call for cooking in small saucepan. You can also use the Instant Pot: Same measurements, cook on high for 6 minutes, quick release.

NUTRITION FACTS:

Calories	327
Total Fat	18g
Saturated Fat	2g
Trans Fat	0g
Unsaturated Fat	15g
Cholesterol	0mg
Sodium	315mg
Carbohydrates	35g
Fiber	13g
Sugar	14g
Protein	10g

DAY 9

Breakfast: SWEET POTATO HASH AND FRIED EGGS

What's better than sweet potato hash? Sweet potato hash with fried eggs! If you've got a food processor or spiralizer, make this breakfast pronto!

PREP TIME: 10 Minutes

COOK TIME: 15 Minutes

TOTAL TIME: 25 Minutes

SERVINGS: 2 servings

INGREDIENTS:

For the hash:

1 large garnet yam I use the term yam and sweet potato interchangeably
1 big pinch of kosher salt
Several turns of freshly ground black pepper
A few shakes of garlic powder
A couple of dashes of onion powder
A sprinkle of dried herbs I used Penzeys Parisien Bonnes Herbes

2 tablespoons fat of choice I used lard
Aleppo pepper optional

For the eggs:

4 large eggs 2 per serving
1 tablespoon ghee or avocado oil
Kosher salt
Freshly ground black pepper
Aleppo pepper optional

INSTRUCTIONS:

Grab a yam or seven, depending on how many folks you'll be feeding.

Peel and cut the yam lengthwise so the slices fit in the feeding tube of your food processor. Attach the julienne slicer blade to the machine and shred the yams. (Alternatively, you can use a spiralizer to make sweet potato "noodles.")

Transfer the shredded yams to a large bowl and toss with salt, pepper, garlic and onion powders, and dried herbs. You can definitely substitute fresh alliums and herbs if you've got them. Taste the mixture and adjust the seasoning.

Heat the fat in a large cast iron skillet over medium heat. When the oil is shimmering, add the seasoned sweet potatoes/yams.

Toss everything in the fat and stir-fry for a minute. Then, pop on a lid for a few more minutes while the yams cook. The hash is ready when there's some crunchy brown bits and texture is soft and tender.

You can plate it up with a dash of Aleppo pepper and gobble up the hash by itself or you can split the hash into two servings and top each dish with a couple of sunny-side-up eggs. The addition of the eggs brings a wonderful richness to the hash, making this a full and well-rounded dish with plenty o' fat and protein to go with the carbs.

Add a tablespoon of ghee to a hot 8-inch cast iron skillet over medium-low heat. When the fat shimmers, crack two eggs into a bowl and pour 'em gently into the hot pan.

Season the eggs with salt and pepper, and cover with a lid for 2-3 minutes, depending on how runny you like your yolks.

Once they're done, carefully slide them out of the skillet and on top of a mound of hash. Repeat with the remaining eggs. Sprinkle some more Aleppo pepper on top.

NOTES: Feel free to change up the seasoning with whatever you have on hand!

NUTRITIONFACTS:

Calories: 574kcal | Carbohydrates: 60g | Protein: 14g | Fat: 31g | Fiber: 9g

Lunch: SHRIMP COBB SALAD WITH LEMON GARLIC VINAIGRETTE

Perfectly seasoned grilled shrimp with crispy bacon, tomatoes, avocado and soft boiled eggs makes the best healthy, BBQ ready Cobb salad for summer! It's tossed in an easy lemon garlic vinaigrette with your favorite salad greens for a flavor-packed low carb, Paleo, and Whole30 compliant meal.

PREP TIME: 10 Minutes

COOK TIME: 10 Minutes

TOTAL TIME: 20 Minutes

SERVINGS: 6 Servings

INGREDIENTS:

Dressing:

2 tbsp fresh lemon juice
1 tsp spicy brown mustard
3 cloves garlic minced
1/8 tsp sea salt
1/8 tsp black pepper

1/4 cup olive oil (use one you like the flavor of since it will come through!

salad:

1 lb shrimp peeled and deveined
Primal palate sea food seasoning OR salt and pepper to season shrimp
1 tbsp organic coconut oil or rendered bacon fat to brush on grill or grill pan
6-8 slices nitrate free bacon cooked and crumbled (use sugar free for Whole30)
3 large eggs soft boiled (see instructions)
3/4 cup cherry tomatoes halved
1 ripe avocado
5 oz container baby spinach or your favorite salad greens
Thinly sliced chives or scallions for garnish

INSTRUCTIONS:

Dressing:

Place all ingredients in a tall narrow container and blend with an immersion blender.

Alternatively, you can use a regular blender (or hand whisk) to combine all ingredients EXCEPT the oil, and then slowly stream in the oil while continuing to blend. The consistency should be somewhat thick and the color creamy.

Have all ingredients ready to go (including cooked and crumbled bacon, before beginning)

soft boil your eggs:

Bring a pot of water to boiling and prepare a bowl of ice water for after eggs cook. Carefully lower each egg into water.

Boil eggs 6 minutes, adjusting heat to keep water at a medium boil.

Remove eggs one at a time with a spoon and place in ice water for 2-3 minutes or until warm.

Carefully peel eggs (I do this in the water, it seems to make it easier!) and set aside until ready to serve.

Grill Shrimp:

Heat your grill or grill pan to high heat and brush with coconut oil. Sprinkle shrimp all over with primal palate seasoning or salt and pepper.

Cook first side 2 minutes flip and continue to cook another 2-3 minutes or until pink and opaque with golden brown.

Assemble Salad:

Place greens on the bottom of a serving bowl or platter, then arrange the tomatoes, bacon, shrimp, and avocado (diced or sliced) over the top. Carefully slice each egg and arrange around salad. Toss with dressing immediately before serving or serve dressing on the side. Enjoy!

NUTRITION FACTS:

Calories: 364kcalCarbohydrates: 5gProtein: 22gFat: 28gSaturated Fat: 7gCholesterol: 286mgSodium: 845mgPotassium: 475mgFiber: 2gSugar: 1gVitamin A: 2475IUVitamin C: 19.7mgCalcium: 154mgIron: 3.1mg

Dinner: CHICKEN FAJITA STUFFED SPAGHETTI SQUASH

When the Mexican food craving hits, this healthy Chicken Fajita Stuffed Spaghetti Squash is the perfect go-to dish! Spiced chicken is sautéed with colorful veggies and served in an oven roasted squash bowl.

PREP TIME: 10 minutes

COOK TIME: 1 Hour 5 Minutes

TOTAL TIME: 1 Hour 15 Minutes

SERVINGS: 4 Servings

INGREDIENTS:

2 spaghetti squashes , cut in half lengthwise and seeds removed (about 3 pounds each)
3 chicken breasts , skinless and boneless , cut into 1 ½ inch pieces
2 tablespoons chili powder
2 teaspoons dried oregano
2 teaspoons garlic powder
1 teaspoon ground cumin
¼ teaspoon ground cinnamon
1 lime , zested and juiced
2 medium sized bell peppers , cut into thin slices (red, green, and/or yellow)
2 medium sized onions , cut into thin slices
3 tablespoons cooking oil , separated
sea salt and fresh ground black pepper , to taste
1 ½ cups Monterey Jack or Pepper Jack cheese , shredded
optional accompaniments: sour cream , guacamole , chopped cilantro , lime slices, and pico de gallo

INSTRUCTIONS:

Preheat oven to 400F degrees. Coat with the inside of each squash with 1 tablespoon of oil and season lightly with salt and pepper. Place the four squash halves flesh side down on a baking sheet. Bake for 50 minutes, or until the squash is fork tender.

While the squash is baking, prepare the chicken. In a large bowl, combine the chili powder, oregano, garlic powder, cumin, cinnamon, lime zest and juice. Add the chicken pieces and mix until thoroughly coated. Cover the bowl and place in the refrigerator until ready to use.

About 10 minutes before squash is finished cooking, heat 1 tablespoon of oil in a large pan over medium-high heat. Add the bell peppers and onion slices and saute until tender-crisp (about 5-6 minutes). Remove from pan and set aside.

In the same pan, add the remaining 1 tablespoon of oil and saute the chicken pieces over medium-high heat for 3-5 minutes. Add the pepper and onion mixture back to the pan, mix together with the chicken, and saute for another minute. Add salt and pepper to taste.

When the spaghetti squash is finished cooking, remove from oven and increase temperature to 425F degrees. Turn each squash half flesh side up and fill each half with an equal amount of the chicken fajita mixture. Top with the shredded cheese and place back in the oven for 5 minutes, or until the cheese is melted.

NUTRITION FACTS:

Amount Per Serving

Calories 563   Calories from Fat 261

% DailyValue*

Fat 29g	45%
Saturated Fat 10g	50%
Cholesterol 91mg	30%
Sodium 480mg	20%
Potassium 1209mg	35%
Carbohydrates 48g	16%
Fiber 11g	44%
Sugar 19g	21%
Protein 33g	66%
Vitamin A 3995IU	80%
Vitamin C 96.1mg	116%
Calcium 488mg	49%
Iron 4.1mg	23%

DAY 10

Breakfast: PUMPKIN COCONUT SMOOTHIE RECIPE

PREP TIME: 5 Minutes

TOTAL TIME: 5 Minutes

SERVINGS: 2 Servings

INGREDIENTS:

1 cup coconut milk
1/4 cup organic pumpkin puree
2 teaspoons pumpkin pie spice (can substitute cinnamon and ginger)
1 frozen banana sliced (omit for keto version)
1 cup ice

INSTRUCTIONS:

Add coconut milk, pumpkin, pumpkin pie spice, banana, and ice to Blendtec or Vitamix.
Blend on smoothie cycle or high speed until smooth.

NOTES:

For low carb, keto version: omit banana and sweeten with stevia or low carb sweetener of choice to taste

For AIP: substitute cinnamon and ginger for pumpkin pie spice

For additional protein: add one scoop of collagen powder

NUTRITION FACTS:

Calories: 292kcal | Carbohydrates: 20g | Protein: 3g | Fat: 24g | Saturated Fat: 21g | Sodium: 18mg | Potassium: 522mg | Fiber: 2g | Sugar: 8g | Vitamin A: 4805IU | Vitamin C: 8mg | Calcium: 42mg | Iron: 4.7mg

Lunch: CAULIFLOWER FRIED RICE

PREP TIME:	5 Minutes
COOK TIME:	20 Minutes
TOTAL TIME:	25 Minutes
SERVINGS;	4 Servings

INGREDIENTS:

1 head cauliflower, cut into florets
2 tablespoons neutral oil (such as vegetable, coconut or peanut)
1 bunch scallions, thinly sliced
3 garlic cloves, minc
1 tablespoon minced fresh ginger
2 carrots, peeled and diced
2 celery stalks, diced
1 red bell pepper, diced
1 cup frozen peas
2 tablespoons rice vinegar
3 tablespoons soy sauce
2 teaspoons Sriracha, or more to taste

Garnishes:

1 tablespoon neutral oil (such as vegetable, coconut or peanut)
4 eggs
Salt and freshly ground black pepper
4 tablespoons chopped fresh cilantro
4 tablespoons thinly sliced scallions
4 teaspoons sesame seeds

INSTRUCTIONS:

MAKE THE FRIED RICE: In the bowl of a food processor, pulse the cauliflower until the mixture resembles rice, 2 to 3 minutes. Set aside.

In a large skillet, heat the oil over medium heat. Add the scallions, garlic and ginger, and stir-fry until fragrant, about 1 minute.

R4Add the carrots, celery and red bell pepper, and stir-fry until the vegetables are tender, 9 to 11 minutes.

Add the cauliflower rice and stir-fry until it begins to turn golden, 3 to 5 minutes more. Stir in the frozen peas and toss well to combine.

Add the rice vinegar, soy sauce and Sriracha, and toss to combine. Set aside.

MAKE THE GARNISHES: In a medium skillet, heat the oil over medium-high heat. Crack the eggs directly into the pan and cook until the whites are set but the yolks are still runny, 3 to 4 minutes. Season each with salt and pepper.

To serve, divide the cauliflower rice among four plates and top each with a fried egg. Garnish each plate with 1 tablespoon cilantro, 1 tablespoon scallions and 1 teaspoon sesame seeds. Serve immediately.

NUTRITIONFACTS:

calories	108
fat	1g
carbs	21g
protein	7g
sugars	8g

Garnishes

calories	183
fat	6g
carbs	2g
protein	6g
sugars	0g

Dinner: SWEET AND SPICY STIR FRY WITH CHICKEN AND BROCCOLI

Garlic, crushed red pepper, and chili paste add heat; hoisin sauce and ginger sweeten the deal. Great served over jasmine rice!

PREP TIME:	10 Minutes
COOK TIME:	20 Minutes
TOTAL TIME:	30 Minutes
SERVINGS:	4 Servings

INGREDIENTS:

3 cups broccoli florets
1 tablespoon olive oil
2 skinless, boneless chicken breast halves - cut into 1 inch strips
¼ cup sliced green onions
4 cloves garlic, thinly sliced
1 tablespoon hoisin sauce
1 tablespoon chile paste
1 tablespoon low sodium soy sauce
½ teaspoon ground ginger
¼ teaspoon crushed red pepper
½ teaspoon salt
½ teaspoon black pepper
⅛ cup chicken stock

INSTRUCTIONS:

Place broccoli in a steamer over 1 inch of boiling water, and cover. Cook until tender but still firm, about 5 minutes.

Heat the oil in a skillet over medium heat, and saute the chicken, green onions, and garlic until the chicken is no longer pink and juices run clear.

Stir the hoisin sauce, chile paste, and soy sauce into the skillet; season with ginger, red pepper, salt, and black pepper. Stir in the chicken stock and simmer about 2 minutes. Mix in the steamed broccoli until coated with the sauce mixture.

NUTRITIONFACTS:

Per Serving: 156 calories; protein 15.9g; carbohydrates 10.9g; fat 6.2g; cholesterol 36.2mg; sodium 606.4mg.

DAY 11

Breakfast: Aip Friendly Breakfast Porridge

PREP TIME: 5 Minutes

COOK TIME: 15 Minutes

TOTAL TIME: 20 minutes

SERVINGS: 1-2 Servings

INGREDIENTS:

2–3 tbsp lightly toasted sunflower seeds (or 1 Tbsp tahini)- if you can tolerate. For seed substitute, use an additional 2 tbsp of coconut flakes or coconut butter (grounded) See notes
2 tbsp unsweetened shredded coconut

1 tbsp chia seed or flaxseed (omit for AIP or substitute with 1 tbsp collagen/ gelatin powder)

1/2 tsp cinnamon
1 tsp ginger, ground
pinch of turmeric, ground
pinch of sea salt
1/2 cup water or coconut milk, more if needed
1 cup chopped squash, cooked (ex: butternut squash or kabocha/ or acorn squash).

If using Instant pot you will need additional coconut oil or ghee and water

pure maple syrup or raw honey

Extra toppings: berries or cherries, pomegranate seeds, coconut cream or coconut yogurt to top.

INSTRUCTIONS:

Stove Top Instructions

Combine all dry ingredients (sunflower seeds, coconut chia, and spices and grind in a coffee grinder or blender until you get a flour-like consistency. If you are short on time, use tahini instead of sunflower seeds and just mix all together. SEE NOTES FOR SEEDLESS option.

.In a small bowl, add the dry mixture with water or coconut milk, let it adsorb and form a gel. Feel free to save a little bit of the gel for topping!

Scoop cooked squash and gel mixture into a blender and blend until smooth.

Heat the porridge stove-top on medium heat just until it starts to bubble. Stirring occasionally.

Remove from heat, pour into your favorite bowl, and top with the dry mixture you set aside.

Optional Add in –>   1 tsp of ghee if desired, helps improve digestion and healthy fats help absorb the nutrients adding in more nourishment.

Top with fresh berries, extra milk, etc.

INSTANT POT OPTION

Peel and Chop your squash into large pieces. Place in the instant pot with 1 tbsp or less of coconut oil. Add in a pinch of cinnamon and nutmeg and sauté for 5 minutes, turning the squash.

Once the squash is coated, Add 1/3 cup of water to Pressure Cooker cooking pot and lock on lid, close pressure valve.

Cook on Manual High Pressure for 5-6 minutes. Allow a 10 minute Natural Pressure Release. Or use a quick release if short on time. Release the lid, drain the water then puree the squash with a hand blender.

Mix in your other ingredients (dry mix and tahini/sesame mix) and a splash of milk (non dairy). Stir all together. Place the lid back on and keep it on warm mode until ready to serve. See notes for meal prep.

NUTRITION FACTS:

Calories Per Serving: 331

% DailyValue

Total Fat 17.7g   23%

Saturated Fat 6.1g

Cholesterol 0mg   0%

Sodium 180.4mg   8%

Total Carbohydrate 43.1g   16%

Dietary Fiber 8.7g   31%

Sugars 16g

Protein 7g   14%

Vitamin C 37.5mg   42%

Iron 4.3mg   24%

Lunch: PALEO BAKED ZUCCHINI FRITTERS

PREP TIME: 15 Minutes

COOK TIME: 30 Minutes

TOTAL TIME: 45 Minutes

SERVINGS: 16 Servings

For The Fritters:

3 Cups Grated zucchini, packed (about 2 large zucchinis)
2 Tbsp Olive oil, divided
2/3 Cup Onion, diced
20 Twists Real Salt Organic Lemon Pepper
20 Twists Real Salt Organic Garlic Pepper
6 Tbsp Parsley, minced
3/4 - 1 tsp Real Salt Sea Salt *
1 Cup Almond flour (100g) **
2 tsp Coconut flour
1 Egg white ▫Olive oil spray

For The Dip:

1/2 Cup Paleo-friendly Mayo
5 tsp Fresh lemon juice
4 tsp Fresh dill, chopped and tightly packed
4 Twists Real Salt Lemon Pepper
Real Salt Sea Salt, to taste

INSTRUCTIONS:

Heat your oven to 400 degrees and line a baking sheet with parchment paper (not a silpat.) .Use a dark colored baking sheet if you have one as it helps crisp them!

Place the grated zucchini in a kitchen towel and ring out as much moisture as you can. Put some muscle into it so your fritters don't get soggy. Add it into a large bowl.

Heat 2 tsp of the oil up in a large pan on medium heat, reserving the rest for later. Cook the onion until soft and golden brown, and then add it into the zucchini.

Add the lemon pepper, garlic pepper, parsley, salt, almond flour and coconut flour. Stir until well mixed. Add in the egg white and cook until it coats the zucchini.

Drop on the prepared baking sheet by 16 scant 1/4 cup balls - or about 3 Tbsp. Press out very flat (about 1/4 of an inch) and spray the tops with the olive oil spray. (You may need to cook in two batches)

Bake until the edges are golden brown and the top is slightly crispy, about 25-30 minutes. Then, turn your oven to HIGH broil and broil until crisp, about 2-3 minutes. Watch closely as these can burn FAST.

Mix all the dip ingredients together and DEVOUR with the fritters!

TIPS & NOTES:

I like these with 1 tsp of Sea Salt, but I do tend to like things on the saltier side. So, if you're sensitive to salt I recommend using 3/4 tsp and then sprinkle some on top once cooked, if you need more.

Please weigh your flour to ensure accurate results

TO MAKE THESE IN THE AIR FRYER:

Preheat your air fryer to 400 degrees and GENEROUSLY rub the wire basket with oil. Press the zucchini fritters out in your hands and then place 4-5 into the basket at a time, spraying the tops with oil spray.

Cook until the edges are golden brown and the top is crisp, about 10-15 minutes. Use a spatula to flip (the bottom WILL stick to the basket, which is why I prefer the oven) and cook an additional 5-7 minutes.

NUTRITION FACTS:

Calories: 222kcal (11%) Carbohydrates: 6.9g (2%) Protein: 3.8g (8%) Fat: 21.8g (34%) Saturated Fat: 2.4g (15%)

Polyunsaturated Fat: 0.3g Monounsaturated Fat: 2.5g Cholesterol: 20mg (7%) Sodium: 415mg (18%) Potassium: 191.6mg (5%) Fiber: 2.8g (12%) Sugar: 2.4g (3%)

Vitamin A: 755IU (15%) Vitamin C: 5.4mg (7%) Calcium: 39mg (4%) Iron: 0.8mg (4%)

Dinner: VEGETABLE RATATOUILLE

PREP TIME:	10 Minutes
COOK TIME:	25 Minutes
TOTAL TIME:	35 Minutes
SERVINGS:	4 Servings

INGREDIENTS:

2 tbs olive oil
1 large onion, diced
1 tsp red pepper flakes, optional

1 large eggplant, about 2-1/2 lbs
3 bell peppers, assorted colors
2 zucchini, about 1 lb
1 yellow squash, about 1/2 lb
8 oz mushrooms
1 tbs garlic, minced
1 tbs tomato paste
2 cans diced no-salt added tomatoes
2 tbs fresh thyme
1/4 c fresh basil
1/4 c fresh parsley
1/2 tbs balsamic vinegar
salt and pepper, to taste

INSTRUCTIONS:

Toss the cubed eggplant with 1 tbs salt and set aside in a strainer while you prep the rest of the ingredients. This will draw out any bitter juices.
Roast peppers in a broiler or over a gas burner until skin is charred. Put in a plastic bag and let sit 10 minutes before removing skin and seeds. Dice.

Meanwhile, heat 2 tbs olive oil in a Dutch oven over medium heat. Add onion and red pepper and cook until just translucent, about 5 minutes. Thoroughly rinse the eggplant to remove salt and add it to the pot. Continue to cook, stirring regularly, until eggplant is partially cooked, about 5 minutes.

Add zucchini, squash, and mushrooms. Season with salt and pepper to taste and cook until mushrooms release their juices, about 10 minutes. Add tomato paste and garlic, cook for another 1-2 minutes until fragrant. Add tomatoes, stir in roasted peppers, and simmer 5 more minutes.

Stir in fresh herbs, reserving some for garnish, and adjust seasoning. Brighten with a splash of vinegar and serve either warm or at room temperature.

NUTRITIONALINFO:

Calories:	175
Fat:	5.5g
Saturated Fat:	0.8g
Trans Fat:	0.0g
Sodium:	71mg
Total Carbohydrate:	27.3g
Dietary Fiber:	7.8g
Sugars:	16.1g

Protein: 6.7g

116

DAY 12

Breakfast: MAPLE PECAN BANANA BREAKFAST BAKEt

This healthy paleo and vegan banana breakfast bake is loaded with maple flavor, cinnamon and hearty pecans for a sweet satisfying breakfast treat. Gluten free, dairy free, egg free, refined sugar free, oil free and kid approved!

PREP TIME: 10 minutes

COOK TIME: 30 minutes

TOTAL TIME: 40 minutes

SERVINGS: 10 Servings

INGREDIENTS:

2 medium overripe bananas mashed
1/3 cup smooth almond butter unsweetened
3 Tbsp pure maple syrup
3 Tbsp unsweetened applesauce
1 1/2 tsp pure vanilla extract
2 flax eggs: 2 Tbsp flaxseed + 5 Tbsp water set aside for 10-15 mins
1 1/4 cup blanched almond flour
2 tsp cinnamon

1/2 tsp baking soda
1/4 tsp fine grain sea salt
1/2 cup chopped pecans

INSTRUCTIONS:

Preheat your oven to 375 degrees and grease two small skillets (6") or 1 larger skillet (9-10") with coconut oil, or line a square baking pan with parchment paper.

In a large bowl, whisk together the mashed bananas, almond butter, maple syrup, applesauce, and vanilla until smooth. Add in the flax eggs and whisk to combine.

Stir in the almond flour, cinnamon, baking soda and salt until a smooth batter forms. Fold in pecans, leaving 2 Tbsp to sprinkle over the top.
Divide batter between the 2 6 inch skillets or a 9" baking dish/pan and bake in the preheated oven for about 25-30 minutes if using skillets and 35-40 if using a single baking dish.

serve warm, drizzled with additional maple syrup if desired. enjoy!

Notes: To make the flax eggs, mix 2 Tbsp flaxseed with 5 Tbsp water and set aside for 10-15 mins, then add to recipe as you would raw eggs.

NUTRITION FACTS:

Calories: 221kcal Carbohydrates: 16g Protein: 5g Fat: 16g Saturated Fat: 1g Sodium: 123mg Potassium: 199mg Fiber: 4g Sugar: 8g Vitamin A: 15IU Vitamin C: 2.1mg Calcium: 80mg Iron: 1.2mg

Lunch: ROASTED BUTTERNUT SqUASH CAULIFLOWER SALAD

PREP TIME: 10 Minutes

COOK TIME: 20 Minutes

TOTAL TIME: 30 Minutes

SERVINGS: 4 Servings

INGREDIENTS:

For The Salad:

1 medium cauliflower head — cut into florets
1 small butternut squash — peeled and cut in cubes
1 tbsp olive oil
salt and black pepper
¼ cup red onion — chopped
1 tablespoon green onions — chopped

For Dressing:

1/2 cup vegenaise or traditional mayonnaise
2 tablespoon Dijon mustard
1 teaspoon garlic — minced
Salt and pepper

INSTRUCTIONS:

First, steam the head of cauliflower. In a large pot add about 2 cups of water and place a steamer basket in the bottom.

Bring the water to a boil. Add the cauliflower florets into the steamer basket.

Cover the pot and steam until the cauliflower florets are tender 6-8 minutes. The time will depend on how tender you prefer your cauliflower florets to be.

Remove from the heat and also remove the lid from the pot. Let the cauliflower cool down for 5 minutes.

While the cauliflower florets are been steamed, roast the butternut squash. Preheat oven to 400 degrees. On a baking sheet lined with parchment paper or silicone mat, place butternut squash and toss in olive oil and season with salt and black pepper. Mix well to combine.

Roast in the oven for 15-20 minutes (It'll depend on the size of the butternut squash diced).

Place the steamed cauliflower, the roasted butternut squash and the red onions in a bowl.
In a small glass bowl, add all the ingredients for the dressing and whisk everything together to combine.

Taste to check the seasoning and pour over the salad.

Mix all the ingredients together until well combined and garnish it with green onions.

NUTRITION FACTS:

Amount per serving (1/4) — Calories: 287, Fat: 22g, Saturated Fat: 1.6g, Sodium: 453mg, Carbohydrates: 17.3g, Fiber: 5.5g, Sugar: 5.4g, Protein: 4g

Dinner: MEDITERRANEAN CAULIFLOWER RICE

Low carb & paleo friendly Mediterranean Cauliflower Rice - make it in 20 minutes or less for a healthy & filling side dish! Vegan + Whole30 + Gluten Free

PREP TIME: 10 Minutes

COOK TIME: 10 Minutes

TOTAL TIME: 20 Minutes

SERVINGS: 4 Servings

INGREDIENTS:

One medium head cauliflower, about 3 cups riced
One tablespoon olive oil
1/4 cup onion, chopped
Two cloves garlic, minced
One tablespoon lemon juice
zest from half a lemon
Two tablespoons pinenuts
1/4 teaspoon red chili flakes
fresh parsley , chopped

INSTRUCTIONS:

Prep the cauliflower: Remove the cauliflower leaves and stems and chop into cite sized florets. Push the cauliflower florets into a running food processor with the grating attachment.

Alternatively, rice the cauliflower using a box grater.

Heat up the olive oil in a large skillet. When the oil is hot add the onion and sauté for 4-5 minutes on a medium heat or until they become soft and translucent. Add the garlic and cook another minute.

Add the cauliflower to the skillet. Stir to mix everything together well.

Turn the heat up to high and add the lemon, zest, pine nuts and chili flakes. Cook for another minute. The high heat will draw out excess moisture in the cauliflower so it doesn't get too mushy.

Remove from the heat and stir in the parsley. Taste and season with more salt as needed - serve warm and enjoy!

NOTES: Optional adds-ins: chopped sun dried tomatoes, feta, chopped basil.

NUTRITION FACTS:

Amount Per Serving: CALORIES: 71 SODIUM: 38mg CARBOHYDRATES: 8g FIBER: 2g SUGAR: 3g PROTEIN: 3g

DAY 13

Breakfast: VEGAN SWEET POTATO BREAKFAST BOWL

PREP TIME: 5 Minutes

TOTAL TIME: 5 minutes

SERVINGS: 1 Serving

INGREDIENTS:

1 sweet potato skin on, baked or microwaved until really soft inside
Sliced pear
Almond butter
Almond yogurt
Pepitas
Dried cherries
Dried cranberries
Hemp hearts
Cacao nibs

INSTRUCTIONS:

Place the cooked sweet potato in a bowl and top with all of your favourite toppings.
Yep, it's really that easy! Dig in!

NUTRITION FACTS:

Calories: 112kcal | Carbohydrates: 26g | Protein: 2g | Fat: 1g | Saturated Fat: 1g | Sodium: 72mg | Potassium: 438mg | Fiber: 4g | Sugar: 5g | Vitamin A: 18445IU | Vitamin C: 3.1mg | Calcium: 39mg | Iron: 0.8mg

Lunch: VEGAN ZUCCHINI PASTA ALFREDO

This Vegan Zucchini Pasta Alfredo is perfect for summer. The zucchini noodles are lighter than pasta but still tasty when you're craving something creamy but don't want the too many carbs.

PREP TIME: 15 Minutes

TOTAL TIME: 15 Minutes

SERVINGS: 2 Servings

INGREDIENTS:

2 medium zucchinis spiralized
1-2 TB Vegan Parmesan (optional)
Quick Alfredo Sauce
1/2 cup raw cashews soaked for a few hours or in boiling water for 10 minutes

2 TB lemon juice
3 TB nutritional yeast
2 tsp white miso (can sub tamari, soy sauce, or coconut aminos)
1 tsp onion powder
1/2 tsp garlic powder
1/4-1/2 cup water

INSTRUCTIONS:

Spiralize zucchini noodles:

Add all alfredo ingredients to a high-speed blender (starting with 1/4 cup of water) and blend until smooth. If your sauce is too thick, add more water a tablespoon at a time until you get the consistency you're looking for.

Top zucchini noodles with alfredo sauce and if you'd like, some vegan parm.

NOTES: If you do not want the zucchini noodles raw you can cook them in a large pan with a little olive oil for a few minutes.

NUTRITION FACTS:

Calories: 225kcal | Carbohydrates: 19g | Protein: 14g | Fat: 16g | Fiber: 6g | Vitamin A: 450IU | Vitamin C: 19.8mg | Iron: 3.2mg

Dinner: MEXICAN CORN QUINOA SALAD

This makes a big batch. This recipe is on the milder side because I made it for a large crowd and wanted to make sure it had broad appeal. Spice things up even more with additional cayenne pepper or chili powder.

PREP TIME: 15 Minutes

COOK TIME: 10 Minutes

TOTAL TIME: 25 minutes

SERVINGS: 20 Servings

INGREDIENTS:

2 teaspoons olive oil
3 cups corn
2 cloves garlic minced
4 cups cooked quinoa
2 1/2 cups cherry tomatoes halved
1 1/2 cups cooked black beans
1 cup cojita cheese feta or romano cheese would also work, crumbled
3 tablespoons fresh cilantro minced
3 tablespoons scallions minced
2 limes juiced

1 1/2 teaspoon chili powder
a few dashes of cayenne pepper
2 tablespoons extra virgin olive oil
sea salt to taste
fresh ground pepper to taste

INSTRUCTIONS:

Heat olive oil in a large skillet. Saute corn and garlic until corn has some brown spots (that's the caramelization that makes the corn even sweeter). Transfer to a large bowl and toss in the rest of the ingredients. Season to your liking with additional chili powder, cayenne pepper, salt and pepper.

NUTRITION FACTS:

Amount Per Serving

Calories 120   Calories from Fat 36

% DailyValue*

Fat 4g   6%

Saturated Fat 1g   6%

Cholesterol 6mg   2%

Sodium 140mg   6%

Potassium 211mg   6%

Carbohydrates 16g	5%	
Fiber 2g		8%
Sugar 2g		2%
Protein 4g		8%
Vitamin A 245IU		5%
Vitamin C 8.1mg		10%
Calcium 54mg		5%
Iron 1.2mg		7%

DAY 14

Breakfast: MANGO CHIA PUDDING

PREP TIME:	10 minutes
TOTAL TIME:	10 minutes
SERVINGS:	2 Servings

INGREDIENTS:

One mango
One banana
½ cup almond or coconut milk
4 tsp chia seeds
2 tbsp natural creamy almond butter
Two tbsp full fat yogurt (optional)

INSTRUCTIONS:

Blend mango, banana and almond milk in a high speed blender. Divide evenly among two small jars.

Add 2 tsp to each bowl and stir. Cover and refrigerate. After 10 minutes give it a stir and return to fridge. Chill for a few more minutes and it should be ready.

Add 1 tbsp of yogurt and 1 tbsp of almond butter. Garnish with fresh mango.

NUTRITION FACTS:

Calories: 247kcal | Carbohydrates: 32g | Protein: 6g | Fat: 12g | Saturated Fat: 1g | Sodium: 85mg | Potassium: 502mg | Fiber: 7g | Sugar: 19g | Vitamin A: 930IU | Vitamin C: 35.1mg | Calcium: 190mg | Iron: 1.5mg

Lunch: CROCK POT PALEO HAMBURGER SOUP

PREP TIME:	20 Minutes
COOK TIME:	4 Hours
TOTAL TIME:	4 Hours 20 Minutes
SERVINGS:	8 Servings

INGREDIENTS:

1 1/2 Lbs Sweet Potato, Cut into 3/4 inch cubes (about 5 cups cubed)
4 Stalks of celery, sliced
2 Large carrots, sliced
1 Large onion, roughly chopped
1 Red Pepper, Diced

5 1/2 Cups Reduced sodium beef broth

2 14.5 ounce Cans Fire-roasted diced tomatoes (I like the ones with garlic)

1/4 Cup Tomato paste

1 Tbsp Italian seasoning

1/2-1 tsp Sea salt *read notes

1/4 tsp Ground black pepper

1 Lb Lean, grass-fed ground beef (I used 93%)

2 Tbsp + 2 tsp Tapioca starch

1/2 Cup Fresh parsley, minced + additional for garnish

INSTRUCTIONS;

In a 7 quart slow cooker, stir together all of the ingredients, up to the ground beef.

Cover the slow cooker and cook on HIGH for 3 hours.

Once the soup as cooked for 3 hours, heat a large, non-stick frying pan on medium heat and cook the beef until ti's no longer pink, draining any excess fat. Add it into the slow cooker.

Put the tapioca starch in a medium bowl. Add 1/4 Cup +2 Tbsp of the hot broth from the slow cooker into the bowl and quickly whisk until smooth. Add it into the slow cooker, whisk the soup as you pour it in. Finally, stir in the fresh parsley.

Cover and cook and additional 30 mins - 1 hour, until the soup has thickened up a little bit.
Serve with extra parsley and DEVOUR!

TIPS & NOTES:

We thought this needed the full 1 tsp of salt. But, if you're sensitive you may want to start with 1/2 tsp and cook the soup. Then, adjust the saltiness once it's cooked, to your taste!

NUTRITION FACTS:

Calories: 237kcal (12%) Carbohydrates: 32.2g (11%) Protein: 16.8g (34%) Fat: 3.8g (6%) Saturated Fat: 1.5g (9%)

Polyunsaturated Fat: 0.1g Cholesterol: 32.5mg (11%) Sodium: 904mg (39%) Potassium: 843mg (24%) Fiber: 6.4g (27%) Sugar: 10.1g (11%) Vitamin A: 3550IU (71%)

Vitamin C: 66mg (80%) Calcium: 45mg (5%) Iron: 2mg (11%)

Dinner: INSTANT POT SHORT RIBS

PREP TIME: 5 Minutes

COOK TIME: 45 Minutes

TOTAL TIME: 50 Minutes

SERVINGS: 6 Servings

INGREDIENTS:

6 beef short ribs (about 3-3 ½ pounds)
1 onion, chopped
3 cloves of garlic, diced
2 tbsp tomato paste
½ tsp dried thyme
½ tsp dried rosemary
1 tbsp olive oil or avocado oil
1 ½ cups beef broth
1 ½ tbsp cornstarch (or almond flour if keto)
¾ tsp Kosher salt
½ tsp pepper

INSTRUCTIONS:

Generously salt and pepper short ribs. I always use Kosher salt.

Heat Instant Pot on saute and add 1 tbsp olive oil. Brown ribs on all sides. Let them sit on each side without moving them so they have time to brown. Around 10 minutes.

Remove ribs. Add a little more oil if pan is dry. Add onions and garlic and saute in all that goodness in the bottom of pan. Saute for about 5 minutes then add all ingredients except cornstarch. Nestle ribs back down in the sauce.

Put lid on to sealed and turn Instant Pot to the stew setting. Set timer for 30 minutes. Once the timer beeps let the pot naturally release and do not open. This is when the ribs get tender. If you use bone in ribs you will need to add 15 minutes to the time.

Remove the meat to a plate and turn pot to saute. Add the cornstarch with 3 tbsp water in a small bowl and whisk well. Add to sauce in bottom and pan and stir well. Get all those brown bits up from the bottom of the pan. Let cook until desired thickness is reached.

Serve with cauliflower mash, mashed potatoes or rice. Salt and pepper to taste.

NOTES:

If you have a different amount of short ribs check the timing suggestions on the Instant Pot site here.

NUTRITION FACTS:

Calories: 49kcal | Carbohydrates: 5g | Protein: 1g | Fat: 2g | Sodium: 558mg | Potassium: 119mg | Sugar: 1g | Vitamin A: 80IU | Vitamin C: 3mg | Calcium: 12mg | Iron: 0.4mg

CONCLUSION

By now, you should be at home with this diet plan that Dr. Mark Hyman, a physician, and a nutrition writer, has advocated and popularized. But in case you're lost somewhere between Pegan Diet in a simple term or what Dr. Hyman was thinking about while instituting this Diet plan, or you're among those who are asking if it is the same thing as a vegan?

Let me summarize here by saying that Mark Hyman did not just advocate the consumption of plant-based diets; instead, he was more concerned about **plant-rich diets**. Hence, he recommends that people should take an essentially plant-based diet together with some high-quality meat-organic, local, and grass-fed, as the case may be.

A lot of persons may also want to know if they can eat oatmeal on a Pegan diet. As stated already, the pegan diet does not permit grains that have gluten. In this category of food are whole-wheat bread, pasta, and cereal. However, those on Pegan Diet can take things like brown rice, quinoa, and oatmeal, at a quantity that is less than a half cup in each meal.

Now that you have gotten the basics about this wonderful diet, it's possibly the right time to draw your meal plan or follow the detailed 14days diet plan presented in this book. Perhaps, you could be among those who will tell their story to others about their experiences.

Thanks for reading! Please add a short review on Amazon and let me know if you enjoyed reading this book